PRINCIPLES OF

ETHICS AND PERSONAL LEADERSHIP

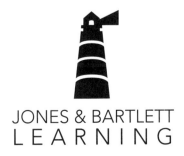

JONES & BARTLETT
LEARNING

World Headquarters
Jones & Bartlett Learning
5 Wall Street
Burlington, MA 01803
978-443-5000
info@jblearning.com
www.jblearning.com

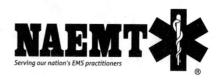

www.naemt.org
800-34-NAEMT

Jones & Bartlett Learning books and products are available through most bookstores and online booksellers. To contact Jones & Bartlett Learning directly, call 800-832-0034, fax 978-443-8000, or visit our website, www.jblearning.com.

Production Credits

Chief Executive Officer: Ty Field
President: James Homer
Chief Product Officer: Eduardo Moura
Executive Publisher: Kimberly Brophy
Executive Editor: Christine Emerton
Production Editor: Cindie Bryan
VP, Sales—Public Safety Group: Matthew Maniscalco
Director of Sales—Public Safety Group: Patricia Einstein

VP, Marketing: Alisha Weisman
VP, Manufacturing and Inventory Control: Therese Connell
Composition: diacriTech
Cover Design: Kristin E. Parker
Cover Image: © Jones & Bartlett Learning LLC
Back Cover Image: © Thomas Fredriksen/ShutterStock, Inc.
Printing and Binding: Edwards Brothers Malloy
Cover Printing: Edwards Brothers Malloy

Library of Congress Cataloging-in-Publication Data

Principles of ethics and personal leadership / National Association of Emergency Medical Technicians, Inc.
 p. ; cm.
 Includes bibliographical references and index.
 ISBN 978-1-284-04257-3 (pbk.) — ISBN 1-284-04257-X (pbk.)
 I. National Association of Emergency Medical Technicians (U.S.), issuing body.
 [DNLM: 1. Emergency Medical Services—ethics. 2. Emergency Medical Technicians—ethics. 3. Interpersonal Relations. 4. Leadership. WX 215]
 RC86.95
 174.2'96025—dc23
6048   2014008024

Printed in the United States of America
18 17 16 15 14   10 9 8 7 6 5 4 3 2 1

CONTENTS

ACKNOWLEDGMENTS

Curriculum Development Team

Scott A. Matin, MBA, NREMT-P
Region I Director, NAEMT
Vice President
MONOC Mobile Health Services
Neptune, New Jersey

Bruce Evans, MPA, NREMT-P
Region 4 Director, NAEMT
Fire Chief
Upper Pine River Fire Protection District
Bayfield, Colorado

Matt Zavadsky, MS-HSA, EMT
At-Large Director, NAEMT
Director of Public Affairs
MedStar Mobile Healthcare
Fort Worth, Texas

This program has been developed by the National Association of Emergency Medical Technicians (NAEMT), A 501 (c) (6) Non-Profit Corporation (www. naemt.org) in association with the International Public Safety Leadership and Ethics Institute (IPSLEI) A 501 (c) (3) Non-Profit Corporation.

Monika S. Byrd, MA
Director of Faculty, IPSLEI

Kevin S. Brame, MA
Executive Director, IPSLEI

UNIT 1

INTRODUCTION AND PROGRAM OVERVIEW

COURSE OVERVIEW

Course Description

Principles of Ethics and Personal Leadership (PEPL) provides emergency medical services (EMS) and Mobile Integrated Healthcare (MIH) practitioners at all levels with the knowledge and skills they need to effectively interact with patients and their families, other medical personnel, coworkers, supervisors, and community residents at large.

The course provides students with a deeper understanding of themselves as it relates to basic principles of ethical leadership and service to patients, as well as awareness of the leadership challenges facing today's EMS and MIH practitioners. This course assists students in identifying their personal responsibility and accountability for ethical decision making and for the exercise of ethical servant leadership for themselves, their patients, and their profession.

Topics and skills covered in the curriculum include personal and professional core values; ethics; decision making; duty to serve; strategies for conflict resolution; and ambassadorship for the profession, their agencies, and the community at large. Through course presentations, dialogue, and learning activities, including written and video case studies, the students will explore the importance of ethics and personal leadership; identify their leadership roles in civic life as individuals, family members, professionals, and members of the community; and practice the skills important to the exercise of personal, ethical leadership.

Many communities are exploring new models for delivering medical care to improve patient outcomes and reduce costs. This course provides essential foundational training that advances the professional development of participants, whether they are providing traditional emergency medical care or mobile-based community health services.

Course Goal

The goal of this course is to facilitate awareness and development of skill sets for the effective exercise of ethics and personal leadership.

Course Objectives

Upon completion of the course, the participant should be able to:

- Articulate personal responsibilities in ethical decision making and the exercise of ethical leadership
- Explain the concept of service beyond self
- Identify personal and professional values and beliefs
- Explain methods of effective conflict resolution in EMS and MIH issues
- Define the concept of ambassadorship in EMS and MIH
- Relate written and video case studies to the exercise of personal, ethical servant leadership in EMS and MIH

Course Units

Unit 1: Introduction and Program Overview (1 h 30 min)
Unit 2: Personal Responsibilities for Ethics in EMS and Mobile Integrated Healthcare (3 h 30 min)
Unit 3: Service Beyond Self (3 h)
Unit 4: Personal and Professional Values and Beliefs (4 h)
Unit 5: Ambassadorship (3 h 30 min)
Unit 6: Course Summary and Evaluation (30 min)

Course Evaluation

A multiple-choice exam will be administered prior to the start of the course. There is no minimum passing score. This exam is diagnostic only.

A multiple-choice exam also will be administered at the conclusion of the course. The minimum passing score is 70 percent. Continuing education credits will not be awarded for scores less than 70 percent.

Program evaluation forms will be provided to allow student feedback on course content and instructional presentation.

Course Attendance

100 percent attendance is required to obtain continuing education credit.

SEQUENCE OF EVENTS

Unit 1: Introduction and Program Overview
- Precourse assessment
- Introductions
- History
- Syllabus (pp. 3–4)

Unit 2: Personal Responsibilities for Ethics in EMS and Mobile Integrated Healthcare
- Reading: Notes on Nursing: What It Is, and What It Is Not
- Reading: Focusing on Patient Care
- Video Case Study: *Sister Act*
- Group Activity: Ethical Scenarios
- Reflection on Exercising Leadership: Personal Responsibilities

Unit 3: Service Beyond Self
- Reading: What Makes a Leader a Leader? A Way Out of the Definition Maze
- Video Case Study: *The Guardian*
- Group Activity: Focus on the Mission and Strengthen the Foundations
- Group Activity: Definition Maze
- Reflection on Exercising Leadership: Service Beyond Self

Unit 4: Personal and Professional Values and Beliefs
- Reading: Ethical Cultural Building: A Modern Business Imperative Research Report
- Video Case Study: *Game of Thrones*
- Reading: Complacency Kills
- Reading: Approaches to Conflict Resolution: Thomas-Kilmann Conflict Mode and University of Wisconsin Conflict Resolution Program
- Video Case Study: *At First Sight*
- Group Activity: Approaching Conflict with Values-based Responses
- Reflection on Exercising Leadership: Core Values and Resolving Conflict

Unit 5: Ambassadorship
- Reading: Recalling Mrs. Wasserman: Relating to the Aged
- Video Case Study: *The Doctor*
- Reading: Isn't Narcissism Beneficial, Especially in a Competitive World? Challenging Another Myth About Narcissism
- Activity: Exercising Leadership through Ambassadorship and Effective Communication

- Reading: Everyday Ethics: Morality Requires Regular Reflection on Day-to-Day Decisions that Confront Us
- Video Case Study: *Patch Adams*
- Graphic: Model for Ambassadorship in Mobile Healthcare
- Reading: The Making of a Hero
- Reflection on Exercising Leadership: Ambassadorship

Unit 6: Course Summary and Evaluation
- Postcourse Test
- Course Evaluation

UNIT 2

PERSONAL RESPONSIBILITIES FOR ETHICS IN EMS AND MOBILE INTEGRATED HEALTHCARE

Reading

Notes on Nursing:
What It Is and What It Is Not

Florence Nightingale *(1898)* (excerpt)

The following notes are by no means intended as a rule of thought by which nurses can teach themselves to nurse, still less as a manual to teach nurses to nurse. They are meant simply to give hints for thought to women who have personal charge of the health of others. Every woman, or at least almost every woman, in England has, at one time or another of her life, charge of the personal health of somebody, whether child or invalid—in other words, every woman is a nurse. Every day sanitary knowledge, or the knowledge of nursing, or in other words, of how to put the constitution in such a state as that it will have no disease, or that it can recover from disease, takes a higher place. It is recognized as the knowledge which every one ought to have—distinct from medical knowledge, which only a profession can have.

If, then, every woman must at some time or other of her life, become a nurse, *i.e.*, have charge of somebody's health, how immense and how valuable would be the produce of her united experience if every woman would think how to nurse.

I do not pretend to teach her how, I ask her to teach herself, and for this purpose I venture to give her some hints.

Disease a reparative process.

Shall we begin by taking it as a general principle—that all disease, at some period or other of its course, is more or less a reparative process, not necessarily accompanied with suffering: an effort of nature to remedy a process of poisoning or of decay, which has taken place weeks, months, sometimes years beforehand, unnoticed, the termination of the disease being then, while the antecedent process was going on, determined?

If we accept this as a general principle, we shall be immediately met with anecdotes and instances to prove the contrary. Just so if we were to take, as a principle—all the climates of the earth are meant to be made habitable for man, by the efforts of man—the objection would be immediately raised— Will the top of Mont Blanc ever be made habitable?

5

Our answer would be, it will be many thousands of years before we have reached the bottom of Mont Blanc in making the earth healthy. Wait till we have reached the bottom before we discuss the top.

Of the sufferings of disease, disease not always the cause.

In watching diseases, both in private houses and in public hospitals, the thing which strikes the experienced observer most forcibly is this, that the symptoms or the sufferings generally considered to be inevitable and incident to the disease are very often not symptoms of the disease at all, but of something quite different—of the want of fresh air, or of light, or of warmth, or of quiet, or of cleanliness, or of punctuality and care in the administration of diet, of each or of all of these. And this quite as much in private as in hospital nursing.

The reparative process which Nature has instituted and which we call disease has been hindered by some want of knowledge or attention, in one or in all of these things, and pain, suffering, or interruption of the whole process sets in.

If a patient is cold, if a patient is feverish, if a patient is faint, if he is sick after taking food, if he has a bed-sore, it is generally the fault not of the disease, but of the nursing.

What nursing ought to do.

I use the word nursing for want of a better. It has been limited to signify little more than the administration of medicines and the application of poultices. It ought to signify the proper use of fresh air, light, warmth, cleanliness, quiet, and the proper selection and administration of diet—all at the least expense of vital power to the patient.

Nursing the sick little understood.

It has been said and written scores of times, that every woman makes a good nurse. I believe, on the contrary, that the very elements of nursing are all but unknown.

By this I do not mean that the nurse is always to blame. Bad sanitary, bad architectural, and bad administrative arrangements often make it impossible to nurse.

But the art of nursing ought to include such arrangements as alone make what I understand by nursing, possible.

The art of nursing, as now practiced, seems to be expressly constituted to unmake what God had made disease to be, viz., a reparative process.

Nursing ought to assist the reparative process.

To recur to the first objection. If we are asked, Is such or such a disease a reparative process? Can such an illness be unaccompanied with suffering? Will any care prevent such a patient from suffering this or that?—I humbly say, I do not know. But when you have done away with all that pain and suffering, which in patients are the symptoms not of their disease, but of the absence of one or all of the above-mentioned essentials to the success of Nature's reparative processes, we shall then know what are the symptoms of and the sufferings inseparable from the disease.

Another and the commonest exclamation which will be instantly made is—Would you do nothing, then, in cholera, fever, &c.?—so deep-rooted and universal is the conviction that to give medicine is to be doing something, or rather everything; to give air, warmth, cleanliness, &c., is to do nothing. The reply is, that in these and many other similar diseases the exact value of particular remedies and modes of treatment is by no means ascertained, while there is universal experience as to the extreme importance of careful nursing in determining the issue of the disease.

Nursing the well.

II. The very elements of what constitutes good nursing are as little understood for the well as for the sick. The same laws of health or of nursing, for they are in reality the same, obtain among the well as among the sick. The breaking of them produces only a less violent consequence among the former than among the latter,—and this sometimes, not always.

Reading

Focusing on Patient Care

Thom Dick *Street Talk (1988)*, pp. 47–49

Thom made the following speech at the May 1981 Portland Conference of the National Association of Emergency Medical Technicians.

I've been asked to be brief in my remarks, and I will. But let me say that I am very grateful to be honored in this way. I'd rather be asked to address [emergency medical technicians] EMTs than the U.S. Senate.

You probably haven't seen many convention speakers like me before. I have no tolerance for long discussions in smoke-filled rooms, no expense accounts or credit cards to entertain important people, no high-powered degrees, and no desire to be in charge of anything. In our political system those things are all necessary for progress as we understand it; they are the bricks of power.

Each of us comes into life as a contributor meant to share very special gifts—things about ourselves which make us what we are, which make us worthy of a place in time, and which comprise our real value to the creatures of the earth we inhabit.

And what makes us what *we* are? Most of us were given the gifts of an EMT, and they are sorely needed today:

- A loving heart, for a time when as never before, the peoples of the earth are starving for love
- Gentle hands, in a time when hospitals and jails are crowded with beings whose bodies and whose spirits have been beaten;
- Strength of character, in a time when many collapse under the sheer weight of their own lives
- Compassion, in a world whose headlines seem to be metered in grief
- Understanding, in a time which defies comprehension
- Patience, in the face of life lived too fast
- A giving nature. For with every run we make, we risk our lives. One of the greatest rescuers

of all time once said, "Greater love has no man than this: that he should lay down his life for his friend."

I'm a paramedic. That's a kind of EMT. I've been promoted to supervisory roles, and didn't like them, so I went back to the street. I love it there. My gifts are there. Someday I may die there.

"But what are you going to do about your career?" my friends ask me. I say, "Keep it." But some of us have other gifts, and they're needed too. The ability to manage. The ability to finance. The capacity to lead, when confusion is the norm. The skill to teach, and the critical knowledge of how to plan for a future which is both elusive and inevitable. The maturity to handle power with wisdom and humility. We all have different roles with the same purpose—can we remember what it is?

A lot of you brought cameras to this conference. You know that when you look through the viewfinder of a camera, you may see more than one object, but usually you focus on only one subject. You want this subject to appear sharp so your photograph will emphasize it, make it stand out. Even in using a wide-angle lens, which enables you to see more of what's around a subject, you still focus on your subject.

What is the subject on which *your* lens is trained? Is it political power? Political power is a fickle thing, history tells us that. Is it money? There's a lot of money in EMS. But there's not a lot of honest profit. Is it personal recognition? There's some. All of these are easy to focus on. But high-quality care, now there's a tough one to keep in focus. With all the distractions we face, it's easy to forget sometimes about the basic thing which makes us just a little bit different from other service-oriented industries.

The needs of our clientele are seldom flexible, often difficult to define and yet always immediate. In human words, our patients desperately need us.

That need has *got to be* what makes us tick. Whatever our roles in EMS, we should be reminding ourselves of that need constantly. We should *make* the agencies we serve *bend* to that need, constantly.

And in terms of that need, we must make the EMT one of the most important people on earth. To managers. To bureaucrats. To dispatchers and supply personnel. To magazine editors. To the manufacturers of patient-care equipment. To the medical community. To public administrators and to the public. And most of all, to ourselves, each and every one of us.

Editor's note: Seven years have passed since Thom wrote this article. Having served as quality analyst for Hartson Medical Services of San Diego and working as a paramedic, he still feels his calling is on the streets.

VIDEO Case Study
Sister Act

Purpose

To explore the transition from thinking of self to thinking of others as essential to ethical leadership

Leadership Points for Dialogue

- Was the action of Mary Clarence to leave the convent ethical, unethical, or are you not sure? Why?
- What does this clip illustrate in regards to Mother Superior's actions when she sent Mary Clarence to sing in the choir? Was she living up to her personal responsibilities? How?
- In what ways did Mary Clarence's and Mother Superior's actions relate to their personal responsibilities to self, the organization/profession, and community?

SERVICE BEYOND SELF

Reading

What Makes a Leader a Leader? A Way Out of the Definition Maze

Kathy Lund Dean, *The Gustavus Quarterly* (Spring 2013), pp. 17–19

If I were to ask ten people what leadership means, chances are I would get ten distinct responses. There are hundreds of leadership models, definitions, and distinctions. For millennia, we've been trying to understand why some people are more effective leaders than others. With the stunning organizational ethics failures of the past decade alone, from corporations to churches to service organizations, we in business education find ourselves encountering antipathy toward the whole idea of leadership at a time when we most need excellent leaders to emerge. So, how do we move forward with a concept that resists clean definitions and encompasses so many ways of understanding it?

I attended my annual teaching and learning conference this past summer in St. Catharines, Ontario. A colleague of mine asked a nine-year-old attending a leadership camp what "leadership" meant to her, and here is what she said:

Leadership is when you're all playing together and you notice there is a kid who doesn't have anyone to play with, and you go ask him to come play with you.

That child's response is emblematic of the way I have come to understand leadership, and particularly ethical leadership, over the years: Leadership is about *action* that makes a difference, and *character* mediates whether that difference is positive or negative. Our leadership camper saw a solitary child, and because children often see the world with a clarity that conflates good character with leadership, she took action that made a positive difference. Conversely, Barry Cadden and Greg Conigliaro have certainly taken action as co-owners of the New England Compounding Center, but because their priority was financial gain, their tainted medicines have sickened hundreds of people and killed 36, with more deaths sure to follow. Those two men represent the worst in the privation of leadership character.

And what of character? Arguably, we should spend as much time talking about character as we do talking about leadership because it's character that determines how a leader's actions will probably be experienced. Yet we cannot see character without some kind of action as a signal to its nature. I think that is why F. Scott Fitzgerald made no distinction between action and character—action *is* character. Malcolm Forbes said, "You can easily judge the character of others by how they treat those who can do nothing for them or to them."

By seeing what leaders consistently do, and the outcomes of those actions, I don't get bogged down in definitions or arguments about theoretical primacy. Even small children know what leadership looks like in action, without knowing (or caring) how we academics want to define it. So, how do we carefully and intentionally cultivate *character*? What kind of space and experiences embed *character* in our students so that their leadership activities are transformative for and affirm the dignity of all who encounter them?

Gustavus is that space, and Gustavus faculty and staff are exactly the people who shape those experiences for ethical leadership development. In my own leadership research, as well as in my role as associate editor for the *Journal of Management Education*, I have seen scholars describe how to support students in developing the character that will serve them in leadership positions. Educational experiences must help them:

1. learn who they are, and where they fit within a dizzyingly complex global workplace. Successful leaders have competence in reflecting on their successes and challenges, and don't shy away from learning new things about themselves and others;

2. cultivate broadly transferable skills like creativity, flexibility, intellectual curiosity, and tolerance for ambiguity. The global workplace is getting more complex, not less, and change happens faster every day. Successful leaders have skills in self-managing high velocity environments while helping others similarly manage;

3. learn *how* to learn new information. Knowledge accumulation is growing exponentially, so a focus on content must give way to a focus on the process of learning. With some knowledge bases like medicine doubling every 18 months, content quickly becomes obsolete, and successful leaders engage with new knowledge that serves others well;

4. develop an appreciation for other cultures and beliefs, and develop a strong foundation of civic awareness and engagement. Successful leaders model inclusion and are not threatened by people with whom they are unfamiliar. They model the process of appreciation and generativity. Successful leaders realize that "community" means all of us, and do not separate "us" from "them"; and

5. develop, test, and become adept at using a moral compass. There are no comforting lists of what is right and wrong in a global setting, because we cannot count on shared understandings based on similar life experiences and faith traditions. Successful leaders understand moral uncertainty and pressures, and resist the absolutism that comes from simply deflecting difficult situations or conflicting values. They subject their beliefs to scrutiny and discover where their own lines in the sand lie.

As I navigate my way and become familiar with Gusties both on and off campus, I am energized to see student leadership opportunities already aligned with an influential report that details how character and leadership have become decoupled in business education and what faculty can do about it. The Carnegie Foundation's latest research study findings, *Rethinking Undergraduate Business Education: Liberal Learning for the Profession* (2011), have caused a great stir in business academic departments across the globe. The Carnegie report has given us a roadmap to cultivate excellent leadership in our students, and Gustavus is uniquely positioned, with an infrastructure and ethos built on our five core values, to follow that map. Liberal education helps students with learning outcomes critical to sustaining leadership excellence in a global village, because the focus is on the *process* of learning as a lifelong sport.

Since I arrived at Gustavus last summer, I have seen transformative and affirming leadership everywhere. One of the key spaces where developing character and ethical leaders takes place is in the Center for Servant Leadership (CSL). Although The Center has chosen Robert Greenleaf's seminal conception of servant-leadership as its organizing paradigm, the CSL's direction in offering students leadership activities and experiential learning opportunities directly supports a broad vision of Gustavus students as leaders in their respective fields.

In my role of advancing leadership opportunities for students, I work with the entire CSL staff. Jeff Stocco, the Center's director, talked about some of the challenges we face in bringing Gustavus's core values to life: "The last decade or so has been a challenge for institutions of higher education. We have been so focused on attracting and retaining students that we have perhaps been reluctant to demand more from them. It has felt at times that higher education has given up on challenging students to consider the big questions, the tough questions of vocation and service. Students need to craft their own path for how they will serve in every aspect of their life. What will they contribute while here? How will they make a difference once they get out into the world?"

It is within that question of *service* that Gustavus may uniquely deliver on the promise of the Carnegie report for transformative leadership education and character development. The notion of "leader" now must include engaging with community and recognizing our common fate with community partners. Developing character that shapes positive leadership outcomes means having students discover their leadership voice, take action in service to others, and reflect on their experiences in iterative, developmental ways. Although my own position continues to

be organic, my responsibilities for helping students see what's possible as leaders include activities both inside Gustavus as well as with the greater community. I have four main work arenas:

1. Gaining new leadership learning opportunities for students at Gustavus. That includes working with the College's faculty and staff across campus to create infrastructure around experiential learning opportunities such as service learning, internships, study abroad, January Interim courses, career opportunities, and community-based partnerships. For the spring semester, my Organizational Behavior students will enjoy service learning opportunities with four organizational leaders in the greater southern Minnesota area.

2. Working with my department members to strategically plan our future. I chair our department's strategic planning effort, and we have identified a host of opportunities and challenges going forward that demand our attention. The department's national advisory board will be wonderfully assistive as we delineate how Economics and Management will best serve students.

3. Harnessing the enthusiastic support of alumni and supporters of the College. It has been a delight for me to meet with so many alumni, friends, and trustees of the College over the last four months. Each time I get to do so reaffirms what a special place Gustavus is for so many people.

4. Continuing my own research and scholarly engagement. My research projects continue to flourish in the major streams of understanding how religious accommodation disputes are resolved in the workplace, exploring what contributes to student engagement, and understanding how organizational context shapes ethical decision making. I am looking forward to

presenting my new work at three major meetings next year, and moving prior work toward publication.

Gustavus is a special place where young men and women genuinely experience who they are, perhaps for the first time. Gustavus is where they have success combining character with leadership, in programs like Gustavus Women in Leadership and its student companion, Women in Business Leadership; Gusties in Ongoing Leadership Development (G.O.L.D.); Career Explorations; and study abroad through the Center for International and Cultural Education. It is amazing to watch what happens when an entire community, both on and off campus, comes together to support the next generation of leaders.

Kathy Lund Dean, Ph.D., is a professor of management in the Department of Economics and Management and the Board of Trustees Distinguished Chair in Leadership and Ethics.

VIDEO Case Study
The Guardian

Purpose

This video clip presents a perspective on the concept of service beyond self as it relates to delivery of emergency rescue services and to the members of the service delivery team.

Leadership Points for Dialogue

- Senior Chief Randall tells the recruit that the only difference between the victim and the rescuer is the attitude taken by the swimmer as they enter the water. What is the application of that message to the MIH profession? How does it relate to the exercise of service leadership?
- When considering your role to the organization/profession, what does the statement "honor your gift" mean? What does the statement mean to the idea of service to the victim (community)?
- Senior Chief Randall relates to Fisch the struggles that he has personally had. How does service to others relate then to the need for service to self? How do you maintain balance?

Group Activity

Focus on the Mission and Strengthen the Foundations
From *The International Public Safety Leadership & Ethics Institute*

Materials Needed

- Tent pole or other long, thin, light rod (referred to as Rebar)

Purpose

This activity provides an opportunity to understand how teamwork, communications, and a focus on the mission are all required for a group to function effectively and collaboratively.

Objectives and Rules

- You will be a part of group whose objective is to place Rebar (a tent pole or other thin, light rod) on the ground to strengthen the foundation of your group.
- Your group will divide into two lines, facing each other, and begin by pointing your index fingers toward each other, at average shoulder height, with thumbs pointed upward.
- The Rebar will rest on the extended index fingers of the members of your group.
- The index fingers of every person in your group must remain in contact with the Rebar at all times, while the thumbs must always remain pointed upward.
- If anyone's fingers are not touching the Rebar or thumbs are not pointed upward at any time during the activity, the group must restart the activity with the Rebar at shoulder height.

Definition Maze

Follow your facilitator's instructions for a small-group activity based on the reading, "What Makes a Leader a Leader: A Way Out of the Definition Maze" and the list of the learning experiences that support the ethical exercise of leadership.

Learning experiences that support the ethical exercise of leadership:

1. Learn who you are and where you fit within a dizzyingly complex global workplace.
2. Cultivate broadly transferable skills like creativity, flexibility, intellectual curiosity, and tolerance for ambiguity.

3. Learn *how* to learn new information. Knowledge accumulation is growing exponentially, so a focus on content must give way to a focus on the process of learning.
4. Develop an appreciation for other cultures and beliefs, and develop a strong foundation of civic awareness and engagement.
5. Develop, test, and become adept at using a moral compass.
   - In an assigned small group, consider how one of the learning experiences applies to your profession and create action items that would support your ideas. List your ideas on chart paper.
   - Consider the following questions:
      - What are the challenges to the implementation of your ideas?
      - How does the activity relate to the idea of service to others from an organizational/professional perspective?
   - Plan for your small group to make a report to the class as a whole at the conclusion of the activity.

UNIT 4

PERSONAL AND PROFESSIONAL VALUES AND BELIEFS

Reading

Ethical Culture Building: A Modern Business Imperative/ Research Report

Research Report (2009), pp. 10–13. ECOA, Ethics & Compliance Officer Association.

Note: Full text is available for download: http://www.ethics.org/resource/ethical-culture-building-modern-business-imperative

What Is "Ethical Culture"?

What is generally referred to as the ethical culture of an organization actually involves two distinct, yet interrelated, systems—ethical culture and ethical climate. The field of *ethical culture* is grounded in an anthropological worldview and, as a result, focuses on the formal and informal systems that influence behavior. On the other hand, the study of *ethical climate* is derived from psychology, and this seeks to investigate the collective "personality" of the organization. Although these two bodies of research originated from different disciplines, both examine the same broad concept: promoting ethical conduct in organizations.

Ethical Culture

Clifford Geertz, a prominent theorist in the field of anthropology, defined culture as "an historically transmitted pattern of meanings embodied in symbols, a system of inherited conceptions ... by which [people] communicate, perpetuate and develop their knowledge ... and attitudes" (1973, p. 5). Essentially, culture is nonbiological inheritance. Parents' genes pass along brown eyes and dimples but, for example, the words and actions of caregivers shape children's understanding. Culture teaches children which behaviors garner social approval, how to react to strangers, whether to care about others' needs or merely their own, and so on. The essence of culture unifies values and priorities that both flow from and reinforce those values.

The literature on ethical culture developed out of the concept of organizational culture, which in turn developed out of the study of societal culture. Like

15

societies, organizations develop their own cultures. In the workplace, everyday actions and decisions are laden with meaning; we learn what is valued and show what we value by our words and our actions.

Consider something as simple as the employee coffee break. In one organization, coffee breaks take place at appointed times, for a predetermined duration, and in a single, designated location. In another company, employees never take formal breaks and, instead, grab coffee and engage in chatty conversation in the halls throughout the day. Both organizations may have written policies regarding coffee breaks, or maybe neither does, but either way it is clear that there is a "way things are done around here." Do things the "right" way and you will be deemed responsible and respectful or friendly and collegial. On the other hand, employees who, even unintentionally, violate the culture may be deemed a lazy slacker or an aloof snob. Such judgments—based initially only on coffee break missteps—can eventually lead to the ostracization or even discipline of the culturally unaware employee. *When it comes to culture, perception creates reality.*

What then is "ethical" culture? Essentially, it is the extent to which an organization regards its values. Strong ethical cultures make doing what is right a priority. *"Ethical culture is the (often unwritten) code of conduct by which employees learn what they should think and do* (Ethics Resource Center [ERC], 2005). The ethical culture of the organization communicates acceptable limits, how employees ought to treat others, whether it is acceptable to question authority figures, if it is safe to report observed misconduct, and the importance of compliance with controls and safeguards (ERC, 2005; Trevino in Soule, 2005). Linda Trevino, a leading scholar in the study of ethical culture, notes that ethical culture determines "how employees understand what is expected of them, and how things really get done" (Trevino, Weaver, Gibson, & Toffler, 1999).

Ethical Climate

Stemming from the field of psychology, ethical climate is concerned with the "collective personality" of the organization. Ethical climate literature investigates the *ethics-related attitudes, perceptions, and decision-making processes* in an organization. Ethical climate includes several dimensions: self-interest, company profit, efficiency, friendship, team-interest, social responsibility, personal morality, rules and standard operating procedures, and laws and professional codes (Trevino, Butterfield, & McCabe, 2001). Just as ethical culture can be viewed as a subset of organizational culture literature, ethical climate is an outgrowth of work done on organizational climate.

The dominant theory of ethical climate was created by Victor and Cullen (1987, 1988), and most research to date has investigated the ethical climate of organizations using this theory and its measure, the Ethical Climate Questionnaire. Victor and Cullen's theory is based on the assumption that *employees form collective perceptions of ethical events, ethical practices, and ethical procedures.* These collective perceptions depend on the ethical criteria used for organizational decision making and the loci of analysis used in that decision-making process. In essence, they examined the answers to two questions:

1. What is the priority when making a decision: self-interest, joint or social interests, or universal ethical principles?[1]
2. Whose interests are considered when making a decision: oneself only, the group/organization, or humanity and society?

By multiplying the three ethical criteria[2] (question 1) by the three loci of analysis[3] (question 2), Victor and Cullen theorized that nine different ethical climate types existed. Additional research suggests five ethical climate types actually exist in organizations. It should also be noted that most organizations combine a number of different climates, and there can also be subclimates by departments (Weber, 1995, as cited in Trevino et al., 2001).

Victor and Cullen's theory is not the only way of explaining and examining ethical climate. Vidaver-Cohen (1995/1998) proposed that the ethical climate of the organization can be more or less conducive to ethical behavior depending on where the ethical climate falls along a *moral climate continuum*. At one end of the continuum is the most ethical climate, where organizational norms always promote moral behavior, and at the other end of the continuum is the most unethical climate, where organizational norms never promote moral behavior. According to this theory, five dimensions define the ethical climate:

1. the prevailing norms for selecting organizational goals (goal emphasis);
2. how organizational goals should be attained (means emphasis);
3. how performance is rewarded (reward orientation);
4. how resources are allocated to perform specific tasks (task support); and
5. the type of relationships expected in the firm (socioemotional support).

According to this theory, an organization with a positive ethical climate takes a socioeconomic perspective and observes communitarian principles. These principles affect and are affected by political, technical, and cultural organizational processes, such as:

1. equitable power distribution, democratic decision processes, and a stakeholder-oriented strategy (political processes);
2. socioeconomic production and an integrated structure (technical processes); and
3. formalized attention to moral concern and an informally reinforced moral perspective (cultural organizational processes).

More recently, Arnaud and Schminke (under review) have investigated ethical culture using a psychological process model. Essentially, this model assumes that organizations form collective personalities and, as a result, when it comes to moral situations, go through the same process[4] an individual would. This model focuses on four dimensions of ethical climate:

1. Collective moral sensitivity: being aware of moral situations

2. Collective moral judgment: deciding the moral course of action
3. Collective moral motivation: caring about doing what is moral
4. Collective moral character: acting upon moral judgment and commitment by doing what is right.

Ethical Culture and Climate: How They Interact and What Makes Each Unique

It makes sense in everyday situations to refer to the ethical commitment of an organization as its "ethical culture." However, as we have seen, ethical climate research and ethical culture research are distinct fields of study. As described by Trevino et al. (2001), ethical climate refers to the "broad normative characteristics and qualities that tell people what kind of organization this is—essentially what the organization values" (p. 308). On the other hand, ethical culture includes "formal and informal control systems (e.g., rules, rewards, and norms) that are aimed more specifically at influencing behavior" (Trevino et al., 2001, p. 308). While there is obviously a great deal of overlap and similarity between ethical climate and culture, these two facets of the ethical life of organizations remain distinct. **Figure 1** portrays how the two interact and includes brief descriptions of each.

Notes

1. Their three *ethical criterion dimensions* coincide with different stages of cognitive moral development as defined by Lawrence Kohlberg. Although Kohlberg identified six stages, Victor and Cullen utilize his broader preconventional, conventional, and postconventional typology. See Kohlberg (1976) for information about the levels of cognitive moral development.
2. Referred to by Victor and Cullen as egoistic, benevolence, and principled, respectively.

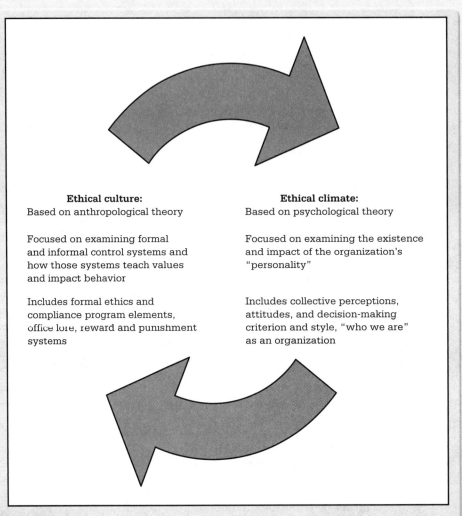

Ethical culture:
Based on anthropological theory

Focused on examining formal
and informal control systems and
how those systems teach values
and impact behavior

Includes formal ethics and
compliance program elements,
office lore, reward and punishment
systems

Ethical climate:
Based on psychological theory

Focused on examining the existence
and impact of the organization's
"personality"

Includes collective perceptions,
attitudes, and decision-making
criterion and style, "who we are"
as an organization

Figure 1 Interaction between and qualities of ethical culture and ethical climate.[5]

3. Referred to by Victor and Cullen as individual, local, and cosmopolitan, respectively.
4. Arnaud and Schminke's model extends James Rest's Four-Component Model from the individual to the organization. For more on this theory, see Rest (1986).
5. The descriptions in Figure 1 draw from definitions posed by Trevino & Youngblood (1990) and ERC (2005). Formal programs include: a code of conduct/ethics, training, discipline for misconduct, anonymous mechanisms for reporting, vehicles to seek advice about ethics issues, and ethics evaluation as a component of employee reviews.

References Cited

Ethics Resource Center (2005). *National Business Ethics Survey*. Washington, DC: Author.

Geertz, C. (1973). *The interpretation of culture*. New York, NY: Basic Books.

Rest, J. R. (1986). Moral development: Advances in research and theory. New York, NY: Praeger.

Kohlberg, L. (1976). *Moral development and behaviour*. New York, NY: Holt, Reinhart & Winston.

Soule, E. (2005). *Embedding ethics in business and higher education: From leadership to management imperative*. The Business-Higher Education Forum, Washington, DC.

Trevino, L. K., Butterfield, K. D., & McCabe, D. L. (2001). The ethical context in organizations: Influences on employee attitudes and behaviors. *The Next Phase of Business Ethics*, 3, 301–337.

Trevino, L. K., Weaver, G. R., Gibson, D. G., & Toffler, B. L. (1999). Managing ethics and compliance: What works and what hurts. *California Management Review*, 41(2).

Trevino, L. K. & Youngblood, S. (1990). Bad apples in bad barrels: A causal analysis of ethical decision-making behavior. *Journal of Applied Psychology*, 75(4), 378–385.

Vardi, Y. (2001). The effects of organizational and ethical climates on misconduct at work. *Journal of Business Ethics*, 29, 325–337.

Victor, B. & Cullen, J. B. (1987). A theory and measure of ethical climate in organizations. *Research in Corporate Social Performance and Policy*, 9, 51–71.

Victor, B. & Cullen, J. B. (1988). The organizational bases of ethical work climates. *Administrative Science Quarterly*, 33, 101–125.

Vidaver-Cohen, D. (1995). Creating ethical work climates: A socioeconomic perspective. *The Journal of Socio-Economics*, 24(2), 317–343.

Weber, J. (1995). Influences upon organizational ethical subclimates: A multi-departmental analysis of a single firm. *Organization Science*, 6(5), 509–523.

VIDEO Case Study
Game of Thrones

Purpose

This brief clip from Season 2, Episode 4, of the HBO series based upon the fiction series *A Song of Ice and Fire*, by George R. R. Martin, provides an opportunity to view the expression of personal and professional values/beliefs in the field, and a situation in which you are challenged by interfering authority.

Leadership Points for Dialogue

- What does the dialogue between Bronn and Robb about the impact of taking the high road indicate about the potential difference in personal values and vision?
- What may be the impact on Robb as he first observes and then holds down the patient being treated by Talisa? Why does he not simply order Talisa to abandon the man as Bronn was asking?
- What does this action indicate about his values? Is Robb in conflict with his values? How might Robb's situation relate to an MIH practitioner?
- Talisa asks Robb, "Then what?" regarding the war ending by the death of King Geoff and he responds, "I do not know." What is the exercise of leadership without clarity of outcome?
- In what ways do Talisa's actions seem similar to the writings of Florence Nightingale? Thom Dick? How might their personal values be similar?

Reading

Complacency Kills

Paul LeSage, Jeff T. Dyar, & Bruce Evans
Crew Resource Management: Principles and Practice, (2010), pp. 27–29 (excerpt)

On Friday night, January 6, 2006, prominent *New York Times* reporter David Rosenbaum was mugged and struck in the head while walking in Washington, D.C. With Rosenbaum unconscious on the sidewalk, an emergency medical services (EMS) response was initiated when someone called 9-1-1. What happened next illustrates the dangers of complacency: An engine company staffed with a crew of fire fighter/EMTs responded to the scene, and after assessing Rosenbaum, they assumed he was intoxicated. As a result of multiple miscues and delays, it took more than an hour to get Rosenbaum to the hospital, and because of poor communication between EMS and hospital staff, it was seven hours more before he underwent surgery to relieve the bleeding in his brain. He did not survive surgery.

David Rosenbaum was killed by complacency—by the "normal operations" of a system in need of repair. Complacency occurs when the organization's mission becomes unclear or is not reinforced and a condition called *normalization of deviance* develops. Normalization of deviance is a long-term phenomenon in which individuals or teams repeatedly accept a lower standard of performance until that lower standard becomes the norm. Usually this occurs because a team is operating under budget constraints or with performance standards that make deviating from protocol, policy, or process favorable. Examples of constraints include system stressors such as a high call volume or a limited number of ambulances.

Often the team or individual perceives that it would be too difficult to adhere to the higher standard when the stresses of the system are present. So, the underperforming behavior becomes the norm even after the stress passes or more resources are available. Normalization of deviance is not an individual problem, and neither is it a behavioral attribute that causes people to take actions that are purposefully harmful. The fire fighter/EMTs who responded in the Rosenbaum case were not the root cause of the incident. If the crew was held as incompetent and cited as the single defining cause of this terrible outcome, the system would have continued on in its current state, awaiting the next victim.

In fire and emergency services, much like in medicine, responders are taught to assume they are dealing with the worst-case scenario and to work backward to avoid missing any life-threatening or unstable conditions that can result in a catastrophic loss. Why was this protocol not followed for Rosenbaum? One of the first steps in resolving normalization of deviance is to develop a more comprehensive outlook of the situation, one that takes a systematic and fair approach and fosters open communication.

Deviations from Protocol

To determine the root causes of complacency, team leaders must discover the systemic issues that factor in decision making. To determine systemic causes of human behavior, it is important to ask why, as in "Why would the individual or team act in a way that led to the undesired outcome?" Typically, leaders must ask why continually until they are satisfied that they have uncovered as many causal factors as possible. Once leaders understand systemic causes, they can start crafting interventions designed to minimize the chances that personnel will make the same mistake in the future. (Notice that leaders should *minimize* the chances, not *eliminate*. It isn't possible to eliminate all factors that cause errors in dynamic environments; teams can only hope to work continually toward improvement.)

In the Rosenbaum case, the patient's closed head injury was downplayed by the EMTs, and they mistook him for an intoxicated patient. The crew's failure to evaluate blood pressure and assess for a closed head injury meant they were not thinking of the situation from the worst-case-scenario perspective. The crew's assumption that Rosenbaum was "passed out drunk" then led them to perform a series of other actions that critically delayed proper care for Rosenbaum. In retrospect, these decisions and actions were deviations from protocol and accepted standards of care. It might be assumed that the crew intentionally deviated from protocol, knowing the outcome could be fatal, but that assumption would likely be wrong and might also prevent the organization from performing a deeper analysis.

The crew that responded to the 9-1-1 call for Rosenbaum typically encountered several intoxicated patients each shift, and the demand for ambulances in their busy EMS system influenced their decision process. The crew's decision to interpret the situation as a low-severity incident may have been a complacent response. Again, this is not intentional behavior; it's automatic and practiced. To fight complacency team leaders can call attention to the biases personnel develop regarding frequently seen patients and remind personnel through the use of stories (outcomes that are rich in detail) what can happen if they become complacent. This type of organizational intervention, when mixed with an open communication model such as [Crew Resource Management] CRM, can work very well to reduce complacency.

For example, for a number of reasons, it is not uncommon for EMS personnel to become complacent and to miss important cues related to a patient's condition. However, if an individual is part of a team that uses an effective communication model such as CRM, some protection against complacency is offered. CRM relies on all team members to provide input, inquire, and challenge each other. In a healthy CRM environment, complacency is uncommon.

One decision the engine crew made was to determine that the patient was not critically injured.

Another was to order a nonemergency transport ambulance. This second decision, of course, was based on the first assumption. How could this occur? Leaders must again ask why: Why order a nonemergency ambulance? Perhaps an organizational story led them to this decision.

As mentioned earlier, the Washington, D.C., EMS system is extremely busy, and ambulances are in high demand. Perhaps in a previous case the EMT-Basic crew members ordered Advanced Life Support Paramedic ambulances to respond on an emergent basis to an unconscious patient. The unconscious patient, however, turned out to be intoxicated. What story is created from such an incident? Someone redirected critical resources to the side of a drunk. This story becomes a cultural barrier against taking emergent action for suspected drunks, and it also helps reinforce the bias that Rosenbaum's situation was not an emergency.

When younger team members are influenced to deviate from protocol or standards by veteran crew members, it is termed *veteran's bias*. Veterans' decisions, as discussed in the last chapter, often are driven by positive or negative organizational stories. Veteran's bias commonly occurs in front-loaded EMS systems that use engine companies as first responders to screen patients for transport. The culture can become such that the patients must prove to the crew that they are sick and require an ambulance. This, again, is a system problem, not one that can be corrected by punishing the field operators.

Establishing and Losing Trust

After the Rosenbaum incident was analyzed from many sides and by multiple parties, the various causal factors became fairly well understood. In this particular case, a lawsuit led to a comprehensive settlement agreement and a host of system changes that were necessary. When organizations harm someone, they owe that person or his or her representatives a settlement—not to make them whole, but to acknowledge the loss and help with future hardship.

More important than money, they owe the person the truth, an apology, a comprehensive analysis of the system that caused the failure, and a promise to implement substantive actions to improve the system. Only this type of response allows organizations to build trust with the public, and only through trust can teams focus on the failures of the system and not the individual.

In the Rosenbaum case, however, trust was not easily gained. The initial comments made by senior authorities gave the public reason to question whether the agency really wanted to understand what happened, or whether it was more interested in making excuses and covering up mistakes. At first, the public was told "at no time did he [Rosenbaum] present symptoms or detectable injuries that would cause first responders to request the addition of advanced life support resources." But, according to the facts of the case, on arrival the crew assessed Rosenbaum and assigned him a Glasgow Coma Scale (GCS) rating of 6. This rating system ranges from GCS-3, which identifies the patient as completely comatose, to GCS-15, which identifies the patient as awake and fully oriented. In most systems, a rating of lower than GCS-8 is an indication to provide advanced airway treatment and place a breathing tube down the patient's trachea.

The initial report concluded, "Our operational review indicates that appropriate measures were taken and EMS providers met all standards of care as outlined in our protocols." That may have indeed been the case. However, if the crew met all standards of care as outlined in the protocols, and the death was preventable, then mustn't there be a system problem? Public trust could have been established in this case if the agency had issued a response that accepted responsibility for the undesired outcome and promised to make an all-out effort to understand the human errors involved. The agency did not do this.

These types of cases are the crucible in which a just culture is validated and culturally accepted within an agency. Unfortunately, for many organizations they are opportunities lost.

APPROACHES TO CONFLICT RESOLUTION

Overviews of two models for dealing with conflict follow.

The Thomas–Kilmann Conflict Resolution Mode is the first example of a model for dealing with conflict (**Figure 2**). The model includes five different approaches to resolving conflict. Each approach involves varying amounts of two dimensions of action: assertiveness and cooperativeness (Thomas & Kilmann, 1974, 2002):

- Competing: assertive and uncooperative
- Accommodating: unassertive and cooperative
- Avoiding: unassertive and uncooperative
- Collaborating: assertive and cooperative
- Compromising: intermediate assertiveness and cooperativeness

Employing the model involves determining which approach is the best approach for different conflicts based upon the circumstances and the desired outcome.

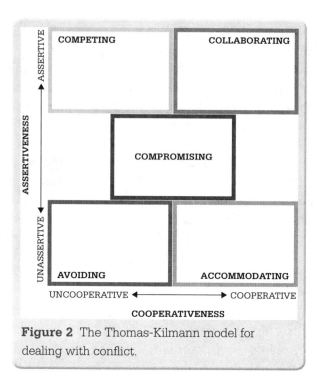

Figure 2 The Thomas-Kilmann model for dealing with conflict.

The University of Wisconsin Conflict Resolution Program is the second model for dealing with conflict. It identifies eight steps that can aid in preparing for and seeking to resolve conflict:

1. Know thy self and take care of self.
   a. Know your existing biases, perceptions, and assumptions.
   b. Recognize your emotional state and what may be your trigger points on the issue.
   c. Keep healthy: Do not go into a conflict process tired, hungry, etc.
2. Clarify personal needs threatened by the dispute.
   a. Know what your desired outcome is.
   b. What is your best alternative to a negotiated agreement (BATNA)?
   c. What is the worst alternative to a negotiated agreement (WATNA)?
   d. What is my least-desired alternative to a negotiated agreement (MLATNA)?
3. Identify a safe place for negotiation.
   a. An agreed-upon safe environment for all concerned
   b. Agreed-upon time and ground rules
   c. Is a neutral third party needed to achieve dialogue and maintain a negotiations environment?
4. Take a listening stance into the interaction.
   a. Actively listen and do not just hear.
   b. Use exploratory questions to gain understanding—seek first to understand before being understood (Prayer of St. Francis).

5. Assert your needs clearly and specifically.
   a. Communicate in an "I" manner. Own what you say.
   b. Be specific in your communication processes.
6. Approach problem-solving with flexibility.
   a. Seek to clarify and agree upon exactly what the issue or problem truly is.
   b. Use multiple techniques to find possible solutions (brainstorming, nominal group process).
   c. Defer judgment on a given solution until it has been fully vetted.
   d. Agree upon decision-making criteria.
   e. Be patient and flexible in your approach.
7. Manage impasses with calm, patience, and respect.
   a. Recognize the need to take breaks at times and "clear" your head.
   b. Clarify your feelings internally and externally.
   c. Keep a focus on the desired outcome.
   d. Maintain clarity of the issue or problem.
8. Build an agreement that works.
   a. Consider the elements needed to make this a workable and defendable decision.
   b. Seek agreement on how to implement and evaluate the chosen solution.

Reference Cited

Modified and reproduced by special permission of the Publisher, CPP, Inc., Mountain View, CA 94043 from the Thomas-Kilmann Conflict Mode Instrument by Kenneth W. Thomas and Ralph H. Kilmann, Copyright 1974, 2002 by CPP, Inc. All rights reserved. Further reproduction is prohibited without the Publisher's written consent.

8 Steps: Overview from Steps for Conflict Resolution, created by Harry Webne-Behrman; found at https://www.ohrd.wisc.edu/home/HideATab/ FullyPreparedtoManage/ConflictResolution/tabid/297/Default.aspx. Reprinted by permission of Harry Webne-Behrman, University of Wisconsin-Madison.

VIDEO Case Study
At First Sight

Purpose

This video case study provides an opportunity to examine conflict caused by differing values and beliefs, assumptions, and prior history unknown to all parties.

Leadership Points for Dialogue

- Why does Virgil react to Amy's proposal the way that he does?
- Whose fault is the conflict and why do you think so?
- What changes after Amy's conversation with Virgil's sister? Why?

AMBASSADORSHIP

Reading

Recalling Mrs. Wasserman: Relating to the Aged

Thom Dick *Street Talk* (1988), pp. 87–90

Remember Mrs. Wasserman? We must have transferred her a thousand times between Big Valley Convalescent and Bayside Community. How could any EMT forget that scratchy voice, so heavily accented you could barely understand the words, or that little body, all crooked and reeking of urine?

And the nurses at Big Valley Con, treating you as though you were some kind of corpse handler, every time you were called to "move 317a." Kind of made you want to quit sometimes, didn't it?

Little wonder that so many EMTs, thoroughly competent and caring though they may be, look upon convalescent transfers with a cold shoulder and a whole dialect of cynical terminology.

Possibly we all could find it easier to care about those pitiful creatures if there were some way to become more interested in them—to better perceive their dignity—to see ourselves as making a difference to them.

Maybe there is.

Did you know that Mrs. Wasserman was a prisoner at Auschwitz for two years?

She was, and her husband died in an air raid in France, although she didn't find out until she had searched eight years for him after the war. Her four children died in three separate concentration camps while she prayed for them, wondering about the whereabouts of the last one until 1958.

Mrs. Wasserman was 36 years old when the war ended. She was a beautiful woman at one time, and her life was spared in prison because her male captors were able to overlook her Jewish ancestry.

She was descended from German royalty, did you know that? Her husband was a Swiss watchmaker, and she gave up her inheritance to elope with him when they were 19.

It seems such a shame that she had to die as she did—alone, a ward of the state. Such a pity, that after a life of so much pain she couldn't have found some tenderness at the end.

How did we learn so much about her? One day Munson and I were moving her to the hospital for some X-rays after she had fallen out of bed, and I was making small talk in the back of the ambulance. Not really expecting an answer, I asked where she was born.

It seemed as though she really wanted someone to ask that question, or any question. She was a little difficult to understand, but she told us the whole story then, in the back of Unit 88, and the things she said changed my life.

When she died there was no funeral, so we sent flowers to the coroner's office in her name, with no return address.

As EMTs, we ask our patients a few questions: "What seems to be the problem?" or "Do you have any heart problems?" Perhaps, if we were to seek more answers of a personal nature, we would find that the world is full of Mrs. Wassermans.

Oh, their names are all different, and not all of them will even be able to answer. But every patient you see has a story, and the old ones have had the opportunity to learn much about life. And because you've been called to treat them, each one can serve as a reminder of your exceedingly good fortune in this life.

Some of them have broken hips, some broken brains or livers, some broken hearts or shattered dreams. Some aren't even old. And did you ever really think about what it would mean to be sightless or deaf, or unable to move your limbs?

Mrs. Wasserman is gone forever. But the memory of her has changed the way we treat a lot of patients. We listen—more than we talk—to Mr. Bolton, the builder of great pipe organs; to May Carlisle, daughter and granddaughter of slaves; to a world-famous architect, the grandson of a hangman; to a pioneer aviator; a newspaper magnate; a murderer; a movie star; and countless others whose lives touch us for a moment in time.

Each patient can help you to perceive the dignity of the next, whatever their appearances. Each one desperately needs your gentleness, as much or more than your ABCs, IVs, or electronic tricks. Each one is a part of your life, and of all life.

And each one will die, Life-Saver, just as you will. In whose arms will you be then?

VIDEO Case Study
The Doctor

Purpose

This video case study provides an opportunity to observe the outcomes resulting from the verbal and nonverbal communication among healthcare professionals.

Leadership Points for Dialogue

- What is the desired result from an exchange between a patient and a healthcare professional? How does the result of the exchange in the video clip compare to the desired outcome?
- What is missing from the exchange between the patient and the doctor?
- What verbal and nonverbal elements are occurring that should not be present?

Reading

Isn't Narcissism Beneficial, Especially in a Competitive World? Challenging Another Myth About Narcissism

Jean M. Twenge and W. Keith Campbell
The Narcissism Epidemic (2010) (excerpt)

Listen in on conversations these days, and a word you'll hear a lot is competitive. ("It's so competitive now." "If we do that we won't be competitive.") Sometimes it's even used as an adjective to describe style and quality ("Hey, that suit is competitive.") People talk about competition for jobs, for getting into college, in sports. There's worry that the United States won't be able to compete in a global economy, and that good-paying jobs will be outsourced, downsized, or otherwise canned. In some neighborhoods, winning and competing are emphasized beginning at age two, when parents try to get children into the best private preschools. Some parents start even earlier by buying Baby Einstein videos or playing classical music to fetuses presumably listening in pregnant bellies.

By high school, the emphasis on winning has reached a fever pitch. The competition for college admissions has grown so fierce that some students spend their high school years on a constant treadmill of Advanced Placement courses, SAT test prep sessions, and meetings with privately hired consultants, costing up to $40,000, who help them craft the perfect application essay. Even some state universities now reject three-fourths of their applicants. Some parents "help" their kids compete by doing their homework and projects for them, even through college. Doctors report that they are seeing more and more repetitive stress injuries among younger and younger children as kids play one sport longer and much more intensely than in the casual pickup games of generations past. Parents fight with one another at children's sports games; in 2000, one father beat another to death at a kids' hockey practice.

In a convenient combination of the American core cultural values of self-admiration and competition, many people believe that always putting yourself first is necessary to compete. If it can help us get ahead, we're interested, and if it's something fun like self-admiration, sign us up. "Show me someone without an ego," opined Donald Trump, "and I'll show you a loser."

When our study on narcissism over the generations was covered in the press in 2007 and 2008, a large number of people responded by saying that narcissism was necessary, especially in an increasingly competitive world. This is yet another example of our culture's blurred distinction between self-worth and narcissism, and the increasing acceptance of doing whatever it takes to get ahead. A University of Michigan student wrote online, "The people conducting this research didn't have to deal with the amount of competition we face daily. We have to be confident and focused on ourselves in order to succeed. So if our generation seems a little more obsessed with the 'Me' than those before us, it is not our fault." San Diego State junior Camille Clasby wrote in the *Daily Aztec*, "Today's college students have more pressure and stress put on them than in past years. The way we're able to meet and exceed the challenges we face is by believing in ourselves. Feeling special is a great form of motivation." Lauren, 27 and from Atlanta, wrote in a *New York Times* comments section, "Aren't self-confidence and belief in oneself basic requirements for success in one's personal and professional life? If that's the definition of a narcissist, proud to be one. And a successful one, at that ;)."

Mike Nolan, a Purdue University engineering student, was even more direct in the *Exponent*. "The country I've grown up in rewards individuals who 'grab life by the balls,'" he wrote. "So for all you psychologists that believe this is some kind of mental disorder, perhaps you should take the stick-up-your-ass-ism inventory and then go cry about something stupid. Mike Nolan, for one, is going to continue working to achieve big things."

Some educators also agreed that self-admiration and even narcissism are necessary for success. "We have a society in which narcissistic behavior is a good quality to have," said Marc Flacks, a professor of sociology at California State University, Long Beach interviewed in the *Los Angeles Times*. "This is a bottom-line society, so students are smart to seek the most direct route to the bottom line. If you don't have a me-first attitude, you won't succeed." Bob Pormoy, director of counseling and psychological services at the University of Nebraska at Lincoln, noted in the *Lincoln Journal Star*, "In this country, the idea of valuing oneself is critical to success. And to me, that's healthy narcissism." All of these well-intentioned folks take it for granted that a high level of self-confidence, even narcissism, leads to success. There's only one thing wrong with this popular, pervasive, and deeply rooted belief: it's not true.

Narcissism and Success

Narcissists love to win, but in most settings they aren't that great at actually winning. For example, college students with inflated views of themselves (who think they are better than they actually are) make poorer grades the longer they are in college. They are also more likely to drop out. In another study, students who flunked an introductory psychology course had by far the highest narcissism scores, and those who made A's had the lowest. Apparently the narcissists were wildly unrealistic about how they were doing and persisted in their lofty illusions when they should have dropped the course (or perhaps done something radical, like study).

In other words, overconfidence backfires. This makes some sense; narcissists are lousy at taking criticism and learning from mistakes. They also like to blame everyone and everything except themselves for their shortcomings. Second, they lack motivation to improve because they believe they have already made it: when you were born on home plate, why run around the bases? Third, overconfidence itself can lead to poor performance. If you think you know all of the answers, there's no need to study. Then you take the test and fail. Oops.

In one series of studies, people answered general knowledge questions like "Who founded the Holy Roman Empire?" They then rated their confidence in their answers and were given the chance to place a monetary bet on the outcome. Unknown to the participants, these were "fair bets," so someone who was 99% confident of their answer would make less money than someone who was only 60% sure. This is similar to horse racing, where the favorites have smaller payoffs (a 1-to-25 pony pays off more than the 1-to-2 sure thing), or football, where there is a "point spread" for each game. Narcissists stunk at this game. Their performance on the questions was the same as everyone else's, but they were more confident of their answers and thus bet too much and too often.

Narcissists also showed their trademark decoupling from reality: they started off saying they would do better than others, but they did worse. Undaunted, the narcissists continued to claim that they had outperformed others on the test and would do well in the future. At least for a short period of time, narcissists were able to live in a fantasy world where they thought they were successful. They were even able to maintain these beliefs in the face of failure. Narcissism is a great predictor of imaginary success but not of actual success.

Narcissists also love to be know-it-alls, which psychologists call "overclaiming." You say to your know-it-all friend, "Have you heard of jazz great Billy Strayhorn?" or "Do you know Paul Klee's paintings?" or "Do you know when the Treaty of Versailles was signed?" and the know-it-all says, "Of course."

You might be tempted to ask him, "Have you heard of jazz great Milton Silus!" or "Do you know John Kormat's paintings?" or "Do you know when the Treaty of Monticello was signed?" to see if he still answers "of course"—even though none of these things actually exists. That's overclaiming. One study had people answer 150 questions, including thirty made-up items. Narcissists were champion overclaimers—they were so smart they even knew things that didn't exist.

Narcissists have a high tolerance for risks, because they are so confident they are right and that things will go well. For this reason, narcissists are successful when investing in bull markets, when their overconfidence and willingness to take risks pays off. In a study using a simulated stock market, narcissists did better than others when the market was headed up. But their superior performance disappeared as soon as the market turned south—then narcissists lost their shirts due to their higher tolerance for risk. This, in part, is what happened in the mortgage market during the late 2000s: both buyers and lenders were narcissistically overconfident and took too many risks. When many buyers couldn't pay their overly optimistic mortgages, the market turned downward, eventually taking much of Wall Street with it.

In the short term, narcissism and overconfidence paid off in spades, but when failure came it was even more spectacular than usual. In the end, the financial crisis was the worst since the Great Depression. It's tempting to believe that narcissism might still be beneficial when leading a large company. Not so, according to Jim Collins, the author of the bestselling business book *Good to Great*. In an exhaustive study, Collins found that companies that moved from being "merely good to truly great" did so because they had what he calls "Level 5" leaders. These CEOs are not the charismatic, ultra-confident figures you would expect. Instead, they are humble, avoid the limelight, never rest on their laurels, and continuously try to prove themselves. Collins profiles Darwin E. Smith, the former CEO of Kimberly-Clark, who wore cheap suits and shunned publicity. In his twenty years of service as CEO, Smith oversaw stock returns that bested the market four times over. Instead of showing in-your-face braggadocio, Smith quietly kept at his work. "I never stopped trying to become qualified for the job," he said.

Collins's study of companies did not originally set out to find a profile of CEOs; he had been looking for company characteristics that would explain business success. But the profile of the humble but determined CEO came up over and over. These CEOs were also excellent team players, something else narcissists aren't. "Throughout our interviews with such executives," Collins writes, "they would instinctively deflect discussion about their own role. When pressed to talk about themselves, they'd say things like 'I don't think I can take much credit for what happened. We were blessed with marvelous people.'"

In other words, Collins found that the best corporate leaders were not narcissistic or even particularly self-confident. Companies with short-term success, however, were often headed by attention-seeking, arrogant leaders. In these companies, Collins writes, "we noted the presence of a gargantuan ego that contributed to the demise or continued mediocrity of the company." This lines up well with the academic research on narcissism and judgment: in the end, narcissists' overconfidence undermines their performance.

Business professors Arijit Chatterjee and Donald Hambrick studied CEO narcissism and company outcomes. In more than 100 technology companies, they found that the more narcissistic the CEO of a company was, the more volatile the company's performance. Apparently the narcissistic leaders were using dramatic, highly public corporate strategies. For example, they might buy up a smaller competitor or start a new "cutting-edge" business venture. When those strategic decisions paid off, the company did really well; when they didn't, it was a disaster. Less narcissistic leaders, in contrast, produced a more steady performance. Given that volatility in performance is considered a negative in the valuation of companies (in economics, volatility is seen as "risk"), the narcissistic CEOs were not ideal.

Narcissists are also not popular bosses. Employees rate narcissistic managers as average in problem-solving skills but below average in interpersonal skills and integrity, two qualities considered very important for management. Another study found that while narcissists saw themselves as excelling at leadership, their peers thought they were below average.

Despite the iffy performance record of narcissists in leadership roles, narcissists are more likely than others to emerge as leaders in an organization. In one study led by Amy Brunell, groups of previously unacquainted students worked together on a task. Narcissists quickly came to dominate these interactions; they saw themselves as leaders, and so did others in the group. A study of business executives found that narcissists emerged as leaders in these real-world contexts as well. However, narcissists' rise to leadership is short-lived. Over time, group members notice narcissists' negative qualities and stop viewing them as leaders. Unfortunately, by then they were the boss and the group had to listen to them.

Enron—the company made up of "the smartest guys in the room" that cooked its books and subsequently imploded—is a microcosm of the downfalls of narcissism. As Malcolm Gladwell argues in his essay "The Talent Myth," "Enron was the Narcissistic Corporation—a company that took more credit for success than was legitimate, that did not acknowledge responsibility for its failures, that shrewdly sold the rest of us on its genius." Gladwell argues that creating a great organization involves cultivating great teams of individuals who can work well together—not just individual superstars. This is yet another reason narcissists are often not very successful in the long run: they would rather take all the glory for themselves than share it with a team.

There is one exception to the rule that narcissism doesn't lead to success. Narcissists are good at individual—though not necessarily group—public performance. When narcissists can receive public recognition and admiration for their performances, they try harder and do better than non-narcissists. One lab study tested this by having a group of students write down as many uses for a knife as they could within twelve minutes (a common test of creativity). When individual performance was recognized by putting each person's name on the board with his or her number of creative uses, narcissists performed very well. When the credit went only to their group, however, narcissists didn't try very hard and performed fairly poorly. This lack of effort with a group will make a narcissist a liability in business, where much work is done in groups and individual work isn't always publicly recognized. But in acting and solo singing, narcissists feed on the glory of the spotlight. So narcissism might be beneficial in a situation like trying out for American Idol or a reality TV show. Notice we said trying out. Once narcissists have to work with other people—which in real life and even in most reality TV they almost always do—their performance tanks, and reality sets in.

ACTIVITY

Exercising Leadership through Ambassadorship and Effective Communication

Knowing enough about your profession's and organization's mission—being an expert about it—so that you can talk to others about it is essential to ambassadorship. Thinking about your personal connection to Mobile Healthcare is a way to engage with what it means to you personally and will help you explain for others the profession's purpose and place in the world. There's not always time for the whole story, however, and being prepared to tell a clear and quick version brings clarity of purpose for you and can reinforce the importance of upholding standards of excellence because the work is important in the community.

Bill Taylor, cofounder of *Fast Company* magazine, recently blogged on *What's Your Company's Sentence?* He relates a story from 1962 about Clare Booth Luce (a playwright, journalist, and Republican member of Congress) and President John F. Kennedy:

"Luce met with President Kennedy, who was, at the time, pursuing an ambitious agenda domestically and overseas. She worried about his diffuse priorities. 'A great man,' she advised him, 'is one sentence.' President Lincoln's sentence was obvious: 'He preserved the union and freed the slaves.' So was FDR's: 'He lifted us out of a great depression and helped us win a world war.' What, Luce challenged the young, impatient president, was to be his sentence?"

Taylor challenges individuals as well as companies or organizations to create a Defining Sentence—a sentence that differentiates you or your organization from all others. There are many other ways to think about this important exercise of describing the essence of something—it is like creating a:

> Mantra (translated from Sanskrit as "sacred message;" often used to refer to a common and frequently repeated word or phrase)

> Slogan (origins in Gaelic from the words for a Scottish clan's battle cry; modern meaning is a phrase expressing the aims or nature of an enterprise, organization, or candidate; a motto or a phrase used repeatedly)

> Elevator Speech

> Parking Lot Talk

> 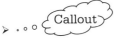 T-shirt Identity

> Callout

> Tweet

What do these things have in common?

✓ They bring clarity, definition, and attention to the most important, highest purpose of a person, an organization or a product
✓ They create positive, inspiring, memorable message
✓ They are succinct; short enough for a quick elevator ride, a brisk walk to the car, or to be easily visible on a t-shirt, or quote in a cartoon bubble, or less than 140 characters

Small Group Activity on Ambassadorship and Communication

_____

_____

_____

_____

_____

_____

_____

_____

Individual Activity on Ambassadorship and Communication

_____

_____

_____

_____

_____

_____

_____

_____

_____

Reading

Everyday Ethics: Morality Requires Regular Reflection on the Day-to-Day Decisions That Confront Us

Thomas Shanks, S.J. *The Markkula Center for Applied Ethics (1997)*

"Have you taken the mandatory training for business ethics?" Dilbert's manager asks the popular comic strip engineer one day. Without missing a beat, Dilbert turns from his cubicle's computer and responds, "No, but if you say I did, then you'll save some money on training, which you can spend to decorate your office." Obviously taken with this suggestion, the manager says, "Luckily, I haven't taken the training myself." Dilbert adds, "I hear it's mostly common sense anyway." DILBERT © 1995 Scott Adams. Used by permission of UNIVERSAL UCLICK. All rights reserved.

The ethics Dilbert is talking about might be called everyday ethics. As philosopher Mike Martin notes, the moral aspects of day-to-day living are "more direct, persistent, and urgent" than the global moral issues—immigration, capital punishment, welfare reform—we might be at ease discussing over the dinner table.

"Why is that?" Martin asks. These topics, he says, "evoke our genuine concern, and sometimes they require our immediate action. Because we lack the authority to settle these issues, however, we can maintain a comfortable distance between us and them."

That distance—and the comfort that comes with it—diminishes when we make ethics part of our everyday reflection, asking ourselves, "How *am* I doing at 'the art of human being'" as artist Laurel Birch describes it? Ethics is intimately bound up with that art because, at its heart, are human relationships.

How We Treat One Another

In *The Leadership Compass*, John Wilcox and Susan Ebbs write, "Moral behavior is concerned primarily with the interpersonal dimension of our behavior: how we treat one another individually and in groups—and, increasingly, other species and the environment." The key here is that morality brings us into contact with others and asks us to consider the quality of that contact.

How many times have we asked ourselves: Is that the way I should treat someone else? Is that the way someone else should treat me? Because we have the ability to be critical of our interpersonal behavior and our contact with animals in the physical world, we have the ability to develop codes and norms to guide that behavior. Those moral norms and codes, plus a set of virtuous character traits, are what we mean when we talk about ethics.

Ethics poses questions about how we ought to act in relationships and how we should live with one another. Ethics asks us to consider whether our actions are right or wrong. It also asks us how those character traits that help humans flourish (such as integrity, honesty, faithfulness, and compassion) play out in everyday living.

Ethical norms and principles have developed over time and across cultures as rational people of goodwill consider human relationships and how human beings act when they are at their best.

In the past few years, I've had the chance to talk with hundreds of people about humanity at its best—and worst—including students, parents, educators, lawyers, engineers, physicians and allied health providers, journalists and television producers, CEOs, CFOs, managers and employees in all sorts of businesses, community leaders and community members at large, people rich and poor, and everyone in between. I've asked them to name the commonplace moral questions they confront in their day-to-day living or at work.

The Nitty-Gritty

Just a few of their responses: Is it right to keep my mouth shut when I know a neighbor's child is getting into real trouble? How should I decide when it's time to put my parent in a nursing home? Do I release software I know isn't really ready? When's the right time to "let go" of my child? Is it right to be chronically late for meetings because I'm busy? Do I laugh at a sexist or racist joke? How ought I to love my spouse in the first year of marriage? In the 60th year?

Despite our many differences, we share these everyday questions; this is the common "stuff" of human living and interacting. We also share a hunger for ethical approaches to these questions. A *Times-Mirror* survey released a few years ago showed that, for the first time in a decade, Americans named ethics, or rather a decline in ethics, as one of the most important problems facing the United States, after crime, health care, and jobs. Ethics and drugs were tied for fourth and fifth place.

Most people would indeed like to live an ethical life and to make good ethical decisions, but there are several problems. One, we might call the everyday stumbling blocks to ethical behavior. Consider these: My small effort won't really make a difference. People may think badly of me. It's hard to know the right thing to do. My pride gets in the way. It may hurt my career. It just went by too quickly. There's a cost to doing the right thing.

Now, how would you respond if your own children were the ones making these excuses for their behavior? Oh, Mom, what I do won't really make a difference. Dad, I just didn't know what to do. Grandma, my friends won't like me. I won't get invited to anybody's home. I know I'll just never date again.

Put like this, ethics seems easier. But we still confront a practical obstacle, much as anti-smoking public service announcements did years ago. Research showed these ads were tremendously successful in getting people to recognize the addiction and want to kick the habit. The problem was that the ads didn't teach people how to do it.

The Five Questions: A Systematic Approach

The same is true of ethics. People need a systematic way to approach living an ethical life. Here are five questions that, used daily, can help with the how-to of everyday morality.

Did I practice any virtues today? In *The Book of Virtues*, William Bennett notes that virtues are "habits of the heart" we learn through models—the loving parent or aunt, the demanding teacher, the respectful manager, the honest shopkeeper. They are the best parts of ourselves. Ask yourself, did I cross a line today that gave up one of those parts? Or was I, at least some of the time, a person who showed integrity, trustworthiness, honesty, compassion, or any of the other virtues I was taught as a child?

Did I do more good than harm today? Or did I try to? Consider the short-term and long-term consequences of your actions.

Did I treat people with dignity and respect today? All human beings should be treated with dignity simply because they are human. People have moral rights, especially the fundamental right to be treated as free and equal human beings, not as things to be manipulated, controlled, or cast away. How did my actions today respect the moral rights and the dignified treatment to which every person is entitled?

Was I fair and just today? Did I treat each person the same unless there was some relevant moral reason to treat him or her differently? Justice requires that we be fair in the way we distribute benefits and burdens. Whom did I benefit and whom did I burden? How did I decide?

Was my community better because I was in it? Was I better because I was in my community? Consider your primary community, however you define it—neighborhood, apartment building, family, company, church, etc. Now ask yourself, was I able to get beyond my own interests to make that community stronger? Was I able to draw on my community's strengths to help me in my own process of becoming more human?

From Everyday Ethics to Moral Leadership

This everyday ethical reflection must occur before we can effectively confront the larger moral questions. A person who wants to take moral leadership on global issues must, according to author Parker Palmer, "take special responsibility for what's going on inside his or her own self, inside his or her own consciousness, lest the act of leadership create more harm than good."

Palmer goes on to suggest that all of us can be leaders for good; the choice is ours:

> We share a responsibility for creating the external world by projecting either a spirit of light or a spirit of shadow on that which is other than us. We project either a spirit of hope or a spirit of despair….We have a choice about what we are going to project, and in that choice we help create the world that is.

Thomas Shanks, S.J., is executive director of the Markkula Center for Applied Ethics and is currently working on a book about workplace ethics.

Further Reading

Halberstam, J. (1993). *Everyday ethics: Inspired solutions to real-life dilemmas*. New York, NY: Penguin Books.

Martin, M. W. (1995). *Everyday morality: An introduction to applied ethics*, 2nd ed. Belmont, CA: Wadsworth.

Thompson, M. (1994). *Ethics*. Lincolnwood, IL: NTC.

VIDEO Case Study
Patch Adams

Purpose

This video case study provides an opportunity to observe a series of scenes that demonstrate the values, qualities, and skills of a healthcare professional who seeks to be an ambassador.

Leadership Points for Dialogue

- What are the qualities that earn Patch his nickname? What other qualities does he have?
- What values does he espouse when he self-discharges?
- What are Patch's natural skills and what skills come less naturally to him?
- In what ways is Patch a patient-centered doctor?

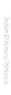

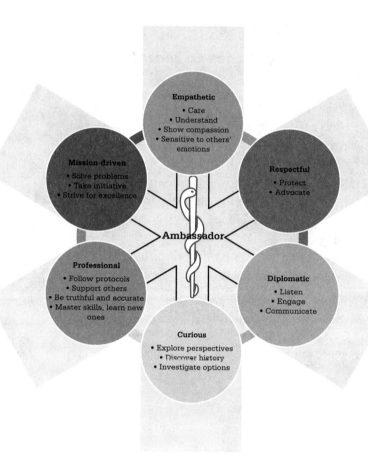

Reading

The Making of a Hero   James O. Page *The Magic of 3 a.m.* (1986)

One of the fire service publications has an annual program of awards for acts of heroism or community service. After they had their annual awards, several of our readers suggested that EMS do something like it for EMS people. While we were pondering the idea (how to do it fairly, how not to miss deserving people, whether such a program would contribute to the quality of emergency care), Associate Editor Thom Dick shared with me another view of heroism.

Not long ago, a California police agency received a report of "shots fired" in a mobile home park. Eventually, three people died and two others were injured, including a sheriff's captain who went to the door of the gunman's mobile home. A .22 caliber bullet fired by the 57-year-old resident lodged in the captain's neck near his carotid artery.

A sheriff's deputy received instant acclaim for dragging the captain to cover, thus saving his life. The county sheriff talked of nominating the female deputy to receive civic awards for her reported actions. For three days, the public recognized her as a heroine.

But the inside story went like this: The sheriff's captain, discovering his injury, never lost consciousness. "I'm shot! I'm shot!" he said, as he ran back to his patrol car and laid down on the ground. A third deputy frantically motioned to a waiting paramedic crew, directing them into the line of fire.

Without hesitation, the paramedics and their EMT partner ran to the side of the injured police officer. He was then placed on a cot, pulled out of the danger area, placed in an ambulance, treated by the paramedics, and then transported to the nearest hospital.

Meanwhile, at the scene of the emergency, a second paramedic unit was standing by. A call came across the radio to respond to the aid of an unconscious diabetic lying in a restaurant less than a block away; the paramedics took the call begrudgingly. "Send an EMT unit," one of them protested, "We want to stay where the action is."

The drama of the shooting emergency went on. Newsmen pushed and shoved, jabbing rescuers with cameras and mikes, and competing with hundreds of spectators for a look at what was going on.

In homes throughout the region, people were tuned into the six o'clock news. "Our helicopter is at the scene at this moment," announced one newscaster, "but we're keeping our spotlights off because we want to protect the lives of the SWAT team members."

Next morning, the team of paramedics who had rescued the sheriff's captain were going off duty. The relief crew questioned them about the shooting incident. The guys modestly described their actions and credited one another for the apparent bravery. None could remember seeing the female deputy who had been the focus of the news broadcasts. When asked about her, they just shrugged their shoulders.

Later, when the press finally caught up with the female deputy, she said she didn't remember rescuing her colleague. The story just sort of died.

As it turned out, the captain's wound wasn't serious, and he wasn't shot again as he lay on the ground, or as he was carried away. Nor were the rescuers who removed him from danger. A year from now, the police officer will have forgotten the paramedics' names: in fact, he may never have heard them at all.

Meanwhile, an EMT arrives at a convalescent home with her partner to transfer an old woman to a hospital. Before moving her, the crew notices that the woman is grossly incontinent of feces. The nurses are "too busy" to clean her up. The woman hides her face in shame.

The EMT reassures the woman and proceeds to clean her up. There is nothing in the EMT's job description that says she's required to do this, but she does it. There are no TV cameras around. There are no bullets flying. There are no paramedics.

"There," she says, finished, and the old woman reaches for her hand in thanks.

The EMT's name is Ruth Ann McGuire. She is gentle and soft-spoken. There are many like her. Their names and their kindnesses have never been published. They are the greatest heroes of all. Obviously, there will never be enough pages in any publication to include appropriate awards or recognition for all of them.

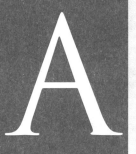

APPENDIX A

REFLECTIONS ON THE EXERCISE OF ETHICAL LEADERSHIP

UNIT 2: PERSONAL RESPONSIBILITIES

Purpose

This two-part reflection activity provides an opportunity for reflection on the content of Unit 2, with an emphasis on considering personal thoughts on the exercise of ethical leadership. This reflection also allows the student an opportunity to identify and commit to acting upon one element of personal responsibility and the exercise of ethical leadership.

Directions

- Reflect on the content and dialogue of this unit, particularly your personal reflections from the Ethical Scenarios activity.
- On this page, write a brief statement that summarizes your personal thoughts and ideas on the exercise of ethical leadership.

_____

_____

_____

_____

_____

_____

_____

_____

_____
_____
_____
_____
_____
_____
_____

■ Use the space below to write one specific personal responsibility of ethical
leadership that you commit to acting upon when you return to work:

_____
_____
_____
_____
_____
_____
_____
_____

UNIT 3: SERVICE BEYOND SELF

Purpose

This reflection activity provides an opportunity to identify an actionable element of the exercise of leadership related to the concept of *service beyond self*.

Directions

- Reflect on the content and dialogue of this unit with particular attention to your personal reflections from the *Focusing on the Mission and Strengthen the Foundation* and *Definition Maze* activities.
- Write one specific personal responsibility for ethical leadership that you commit to acting upon when you return to work.

_____

_____

_____

_____

_____

_____

_____

_____

_____

_____

_____

_____

_____

_____

_____

_____

UNIT 4: PERSONAL AND PROFESSIONAL VALUES AND BELIEFS

Purpose

This three-part reflection activity provides opportunities for you to identify actions that will demonstrate personal values that you commit to acting upon, professional/organizational values that you commit to acting upon, and how these personal and professional values and the approaches presented in the unit can assist you to resolve conflicts through the ethical exercise of leadership.

Directions

- Reflect on the content and dialogue of this unit along with your personal reflections from previous activities.
- On this page, write three specific things you can start doing or do more of that will demonstrate your most important personal values, and write three specific things you can start doing or do more of that will demonstrate the most important professional/organizational values in MIH.

_____

_____

_____

_____

_____

_____

- On the next page, write a brief summary of a specific personal conflict that you are facing; in addition to the summary, state the core problem/ issue as specifically as possible; finally, write your desired outcome and the other party's BATNA, then list the conflict resolution mode that you think will be the best approach to use.

- Use the following space for a brief summary of a specific personal conflict that you are facing; in addition to the summary, state the core problem/issue as specifically as possible:

_____

_____

_____

_____

_____

_____

_____

- Use the following space to write your desired outcome and the other party's BATNA, then list the conflict resolution mode that you think will be the best approach to use:

_____

_____

_____

_____

_____

_____

_____

_____

UNIT 5: AMBASSADORSHIP

Purpose

This reflection activity provides an opportunity to identify actions related to ambassadorship that you commit to acting upon when you return to work.

Directions:

- Reflect on the content and dialogue of this unit along with your personal reflections from the previous activities.
- On this page, write a specific kind of situation in which you think your company (or agency, or department) is struggling with lack of or limited trust, or "an image problem"; state the problem/issue as specifically as possible.

_____

_____

_____

_____

_____

_____

- Use this space to write the actions that you can do that will contribute to improving the situation at your company, agency, or department:

_____

_____

_____

_____

_____

_____

SUGGESTED READING

Websites

Markkula Center for Applied Ethics
http://www.scu.edu/ethics/practicing/decision/whatisethics.html

Ethics Resource Center
http://www.ethics.org

Robert K. Greenleaf Center for Servant Leadership
https://www.greenleaf.org

Institute for Global Ethics
http://www.globalethics.org

MindTools – Conflict Resolution
http://www.mindtools.com/pages/article/newLDR_81.htm

Best Personal Development Books – Values Development
http://www.best-personal-development-books.com/personal-value-development
.html

Articles

Banja, J. (2010). The normalization of deviance in healthcare delivery. *Business Horizons, 53*(2). doi: 10.1016/j.bushor.2009.10.006

Ganly, S. (2010). The development of personal values. *Yahoo Voices*. Retrieved from http://voices.yahoo.com/the-development-personal-values-6418522
.html

Greenleaf, R. (nd). Ten principles of servant leadership. *Butler University Volunteer Center Resources*. Retrieved from http://www.butler.edu/
volunteer/resources/principles-of-servant-leadership/

Heathfield, S. (nd). Identify and live your personal values: Deeply held beliefs and values bring you success in life and work. *About.com Human Resources*. Retrieved from http://humanresources.about.com/od/success/qt/values_s7.htm

Lederach, J. P. (1995). *Preparing for peace: Conflict transformation across cultures*.

Syracuse University Press. Discussion about it retrieved from http://www.colorado.edu/conflict/transform/jplall.htm

McKinney, M. (2000). Choosing service over self-interest: The focus of leadership. *Leadership Now*. Retrieved from http://www.leadershipnow.com/service.html

Segal, J. and Smith. M. (2013). Conflict resolution skills: Building the skills that can turn conflicts into opportunities. *Helpguide.org*. Retrieved from http://www.helpguide.org/mental/eq8_conflict_resolution.htm

Books

Bennett, M. and Gibson, J. (2006). *A field guide to good decisions: Values in action*. Westport, CT: Praeger.

Covey, S. (2004). *Ethics, the heart of leadership*. Westport, CT: Praeger.

Frankl, V. (1963). *Man's search for meaning*. Boston, MA: Beacon.

Gawande, A. (2011). *The checklist manifesto: How to get things right*. New York, NY: Picador.

George, B. (2003). *Authentic leadership*. San Francisco, CA: Jossey-Bass.

Goleman, D., Boyatzis, R., and McKee, A. (2002). *Primal leadership: Realizing the power of emotional intelligence*. Boston, MA: Harvard Business School.

Greenleaf, R. (1977). *Servant leadership: A journey into the nature of legitimate power and greatness*. Mahwah, NJ: Paulist Press.

Heifetz, R. (1994). *Leadership without easy answers*. Boston, MA: Harvard Business School.

Hunter, J. (2012). *The servant: A simple story about the true essence of leadership*, Rev. ed. New York, NY: Crown.

Kidder, R. (2006). *Moral courage: Taking action when your values are put to the test*. New York, NY: Harper Collins.

Kidder, R. (2009). *How good people make tough choices: Resolving the dilemmas of ethical living*, Rev. ed. New York, NY: Harper Perennial.

Kouzes, J. and Posner, B. (2012). *The leadership challenge: How to make extraordinary things happen in organizations*, 5th ed. San Francisco, CA: Jossey-Bass.

Lencioni, P. (2002). *The five dysfunctions of a team: A leadership fable*. San Francisco, CA: Jossey-Bass.

O'Brien, M.E. (2010). *Servant leadership in nursing: Spirituality and practice in contemporary healthcare*. Sudbury, MA: Jones & Bartlett.

Pearce, T. (2003). *Leading out loud: Inspiring change through authentic communication*, Rev. ed. San Francisco, CA: Jossey-Bass.

Spears, L. and Lawrence, M., Eds. (2001). *Focus on leadership: Servant-leadership for the 21st century*, 3rd. Ed. New York, NY: John Wiley & Sons.

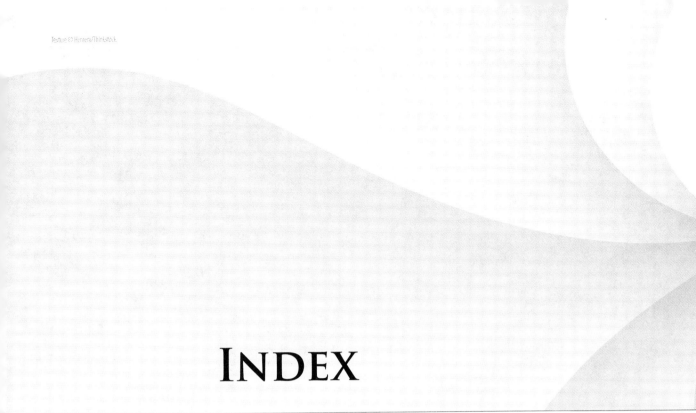

INDEX